Drs. Donsbach and Alsleben

tell you what you need to know about

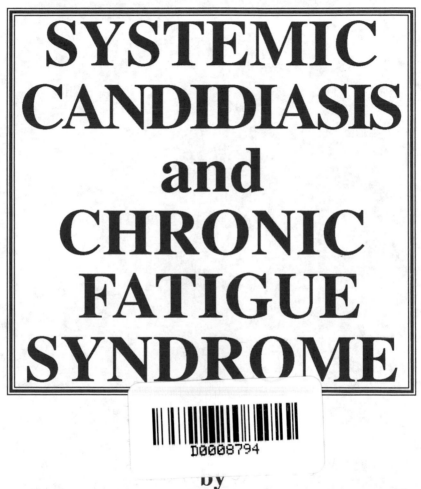

SYSTEMIC CANDIDIASIS
and
CHRONIC FATIGUE SYNDROME

by

Kurt W. Donsbach, D.C., N.D., Ph.D.
and
H. Rudolph Alsleben, M.D., D.O., Ph.D.
©1994

TABLE OF CONTENTS

TABLE OF CONTENTS (cont.)

The Chicken or the Egg?

The never answered question as to which came first the chicken or the egg may be very appropriate in discussing the multitude of new infections we now have in our our society. Increasing epidemics of hepatitis, herpes, amoebic infections, cyto-megalo virus, HIV and other diseases are creating plagues that rival any of the acute infections of yesteryear.

Medical science now knows that the presence of Candida Albicans (yeast) organisms in the body can gradually diminish immune function to the point where an increased susceptibility to bacterial, and especially viral, infections occur. We also know that certain viruses, once they enter the body, can seriously diminish the immune system. The HIV virus so reduces a component of the immune system that bacterial infections consume the body unopposed and are often the cause of death rather than the virus.

Such infections are called **opportunistic infections** because they can only fluorish in an immune depleted environment. These infections take the opportunity of the diminished immune function to explosively multiply and eventually kill the patient. The present therapy of desperately trying to kill the bacterial infection with super antibiotics may be lifesaving, but other infections inevitably occur which cannot be controlled and the patient dies anyway.

Is Candida The Culprit?

We would like to present that bacterial, parasitic and viral infections like Chronic Fatigue Syndrome, AIDS and probably even cancer are themselves opportunistic infections or diseases which have been preceded by yeast-fungal infestation of the body.

We will offer evidence that under normal conditions the **body will readily control Chronic Fatigue Syndrome, AIDS and cancer.** Control of any infection requires an intact and well-functioning immune system. If the immune system becomes damaged, defective, or drained of its vital life-force energy, alien organisms will be able to multiply.

When the immune system is depleted, a prodigious growth of organisms can occur which further drain and poison the body, depleting an already deficient immune system. Serious illness, all too often resulting in death, ensues. **Thus the health of the immune system determines whether Candidiasis, EBV, HIV, or even cancer, have a chance in your body.**

We will explore the following in this book:
What is candida yeast infection?
How does candida enter the body?

What is the relationship between candida and the immune system?

What is the relationship between candida and the Chronic Fatigue Syndrome?

What is the relationship between Candidiasis and AIDS?

What does Candida do to the body?

Is there a way to destroy candida in the body?

Is there a way to repair the damage caused by the candida organism?

In the eight years that we have been aggressively treating Candidiasis much has been learned. We know that the population of candida organisms in the blood stream can be eliminated in less than one month, that bowel overgrowth can be normalized in much less time than that. We know the protocol that will prevent such an overgrowth again.

We want to present the concept that **Systemic Candidiasis can be the initiating infection that depletes the immune system to the point that other opportunistic infections find a fertile field in which to multiply.** We are all constant carriers of bacteria and viruses of all types all the time. They only wait for the right circumstance and environment.

We do not wish to present that candida organisms are the cause of all illness. Many patients come to

Hospital Santa Monica or Institut Santa Monica with a mistaken diagnosis of Candidiasis and we find no evidence of such infestation. The symptoms are similar to many different diseases and can be misdiagnosed. However we stand firm that if candida exists, it will be a factor in every disease which follows because the presence of the yeast turned fungus will continuously deplete the immune system and prevent the normal defenses which would be used by the body.

First we will use a format of facts and statements commonly made regarding candida. This will probably be quite revealing for many readers because there is a huge amount of misinformation about this subject.

WHAT IS CANDIDA?

One must really understand what candida, candida albicans and Systemic Candidiasis are before they can follow a therapy program for symptoms that vary so much from person to person. The following definitions and facts will hopefully present this disease in a way that makes sense and no longer confuses you.

CANDIDA: A genus of yeastlike fungi which develop a pseudomycelium and reproduce by budding. They are the primary etiologic agents for many mycotic (a disease caused by microorganisms, particularly yeasts and fungi) infections in man.

CANDIDA ALBICANS: A small, oval, budding fungus which is the primary etiologic organism of moniliasis (candidiasis). Formerly called monilia albicans.

FACT 1: <u>Candida Albicans Resides In the Intestinal Tract Of All Humans.</u> This yeast is a normal, albeit nonessential, resident of the human digestive tract. It is usually kept under control by another organism - the so-called friendly bacteria which also normally inhabit the gastrointestinal tract. These friendly bacteria, also often referred to as acidophilus bacteria, literally use the candida yeast as food. They also seem to enhance the function of the colon.

FACT 2: <u>The Most Common Cause Of Overgrowth Of Candida Albicans Is The Use Of Antibiotics Without Reimplanting The Friendly Bacteria.</u> Candida infection (yeast infection) was only a minor problem in the years before antibiotics. When an antibiotic is used the killing of bacteria is nonspecific; it literally kills the good bacteria along with the bad bacteria. A very vulnerable bacteria to the destructive force of antibiotics is that found in the intestinal tract, since most antibiotics are given by mouth and travel through the intestinal tract before being absorbed. By destroying the natural enemy of the candida yeast, we allow it to reproduce without control.

FACT 3: <u>Another Contributory Factor Is The Use Of Birth Control Pills And Other Steroid Hormones.</u> Several concepts abound as to just what steroids do to enhance the yeast in the body but I am not sure just what the physiological change is. I do know that most researchers agree that a person using steroids has a much better chance of having candidiasis than one who does not.

FACT 4: <u>The First Sign Of Overgrowth Of The Candida Yeast Is Gastrointestinal Discomfort.</u> This may be in the form of bloating, an excess feeling of fullness, diarrhea, constipation, alternating diarrhea and constipation, itching anus, burning stool, rolling gas, cramping, etc. This in itself is not that life threatening, uncomfortable and inconvenient yes, but not life threatening.

FACT 5: <u>Such Overgrowth Now Has A Chance To Invade Other Parts Of The Body</u>. The area immediately around the external anus offers a fine, moist, mucous-like membrane for colonies of yeast to start growing in a totally new area. Because of the proximity of the vaginal tract in the female to the anal opening, it is an easy jaunt for the enterprising yeast to find a new home, again in a moist, mucous membrane area which is perfect for growth. Thus there is a ratio of over 7 females to every 3 males in whom the yeast migrates from the intestinal tract to other areas which have a similar environment. But we should look at another aspect: even though the yeast has invaded the vaginal tract, it has not yet invaded the internal structures of the body which is necessary for the diagnosis of "Systemic Candidiasis". Vaginal yeast growth creates much discomfort and irritation, but is not life threatening. In the male there is often evidence of "jock itch", a stubborn condition which is directly the result of yeast inhabiting the moist folds of skin in the crotch.

FACT 6: <u>Systemic Candidiasis Usually Occurs When The Yeast Finds A Way To Traverse The Wall Of The Genito-Urinary Tract Or The Wall Of The</u>

11.

Intestinal Tract, Gets Into The Blood Stream And Is Carried To Those Areas Of The Body Which Offer The Right Environment - Moist Mucous Membranes. The female has a relatively short urethra and thus it is easier for yeast to travel. The male often will have the head of the penis totally covered with a white film made up of yeast cells if aggressive personal hygiene is not practiced. A common method of internal contamination of the male occurs after oral sex with a female who has yeast in the vaginal tract. The male will literally inhale the yeast buds and they will end up in the lungs which offer one of the best environments in the body for yeast growth. Another favorite site is the sinuses, also easily contaminated by this method.

FACT 7: <u>Internal Or Systemic Candidiasis Can Also Occur If A Break In The Integrity Of The Wall Of The Gut Allows Yeast To Pass Into The Blood Stream.</u> After years of studying this condition, we believe that this may be the most common method of transmission of yeast to the internal environment. Permeability of the intestinal wall has been reported more and more in relation to allergies and other conditions in the recent past. This could allow the passage of yeast buds directly into the bloodstream.

FACT 8: <u>Once In The Body, Candida Albicans Often Mutates Into Other Forms, Particularly A Fungal</u>

Form Which Is More Virulent And Capable Of Adapting To The New Environment. Now is the time that you will begin to have real problems with yeast. Although this is a foreign organism growing internally, that is not the real problem. Most of the beginning symptoms are because of the multitude of toxins which the yeast gives off during its metabolic activity. These toxins add a considerable burden to your toxin elimination system and also give a constant source of stimulation to your immune system. The toxic overload gives symptoms of fatigue and the overstressed immune system may leave you open to any number of other problems.

FACT 9: The First Sign Of Systemic Candidiasis Is Abnormal Fatigue. This can creep up on you very slowly so in the beginning it doesn't alarm you. You go to bed tired, you wake up tired and you are tired all day. Your doctor may examine you and tell you that nothing is wrong. Your blood tests will probably be so close to normal that your doctor says he wishes he had such good blood. You will go home frustrated. You will begin to have trouble with your spouse and children over little things - just because you are so irritable and tired.

FACT 10: The Second Sign Of Systemic Candidiasis Is Spaciness. Most of our patients describe this as a detached state of mind in which they can observe what is happening to themselves but are helpless to do anything about it. They have difficulty concentrating on anything, even those things that were once pleasurable. Memory retention is grossly affected, decision making becomes a gigantic problem. You feel like screaming "Leave Me Alone!" whenever someone tries to make you cooperate or participate in an activity. You can sit in church or a lecture and never hear a single word the minister or teacher has said - or at least you can't remember it when you walk out. Reading a newspaper is useless because you can't remember what it was you read.

FACT 11: The Third Sign Of Systemic Candidiasis Is Adult Onset Allergies. These usually begin with minor food allergies which quickly become major and widespread. Next, you will be unable to tolerate any type of chemical odor - even to the type of cleaning soap you use for laundry. Perfumes, colognes, petroleum odors and "Pine-Sol" type fragrances are enough to send you straight to bed.

FACT 12: The Fourth Sign Of Systemic Candidiasis Is The Appearance Of The Universal Reactor Phenomenon. You are now so allergic that practically every odor, all clothing except cotton, almost all foods, or anything in your immediate environment, becomes a major problem for you. You are having less and less good days or hours and life has become a field loaded with an abundance of dangerous land mines through which you must walk ever so carefully.

FACT 13: <u>The Fifth Sign Of Systemic Candidiasis Is The Beginning Of Actual Mental Deterioration With Accompanying Delusions, Manic Depression, Suicidal Tendencies, Anti-social And Even Violent Behavior.</u> The possibility is that the toxic overload in the rest of the body has passed the blood-brain barrier and toxins are affecting the brain. This is a frightening circumstance and is the most difficult of all the phases of this disease to treat. You can eliminate the candida but the effect on the brain often takes many months to overcome. This is a tragic phase because the patient often still has a normal blood test and demonstrates the typical signs of what is called "mental illness." All too often family members commit these unfortunates to an institution where they are usually so controlled with drugs that they appear to be mere zombies.

These five signs or phases of Systemic Candidiasis are our own classification based upon observation of many thousands of patients. They are by no means a perfect guideline because the symptoms of Systemic Candidiasis are extremely varied and change from patient to patient; most of you will recognize the five major categories and know where you fit in.

Information And Misinformation

If you are a victim of Systemic Candidiasis, you will probably have gone from practitioner to practitioner in an attempt to find out what is wrong. Somewhere in the progression of the condition a person, be he or she a doctor, a nutritionist, a friend or relative, will have said "You have candidiasis!"

Now the avalanche of well-meaning friends, sometimes well informed, sometimes not, deluge you with do's and don'ts. Remember this is a relatively new condition and even many professionals are not sure how to handle it. The advice given in this book will be a compilation of the experience that both authors have had in treating over a thousand "last chance" Systemic Candidiasis patients at two hospitals and one clinic.

It is interesting that this condition was brought to the attention of practitioners by a physician, Dr. Truss, whose work was expanded upon and popularized by another physician, Dr. Crook. Their approach to this problem was to use anti-yeast and anti-fungal drugs which had a reasonable effect, but all too often only for a short time.

Several other books are now on the market but as more and more enter into the fray, a divergence of opinion can create some very big questions in the mind of the patient. From this comes confusion, particularly in those who have mental and emotional effects from their condition. We feel the following format of statement made, followed by the facts, can clarify the issue better than a rambling dissertation.

Statement vs. Fact

STATEMENT: <u>If You Have Candidiasis You Can't Eat Yeast Containing Foods Because They Feed The Candida Organism.</u>

FACT: <u>Utterly False</u>. Yeast used in foods, fungi family foods such as mushrooms, vinegar and a whole list of other restricted foods on many candida diets do not cause candida overgrowth or enhance an already existing condition of candidiasis. These foods are broken down in the digestive tract to the respective digestive end products such as vitamins, minerals, sugars, fats, proteins and fiber and these end products of digestion are then either absorbed as pure products or left in the tract to be eliminated. They may cause a reaction for some individuals because of a sensitivity or allergic reaction but this is a separate problem.

STATEMENT: <u>Sugar Feeds The Candida And Will Bring It Back Even If You Have Destroyed The Org-</u>

anism Through Therapy.

FACT: Partially True. While it is true that sugar feeds the yeast growth, it does not necessarily mean that anything that contains some form of what will eventually be sugar is bad. Starches are all broken down to sugar in the tract much slower than if you drank a glass of orange juice which has a rapid sugar release. Both foods furnish the body with its preferred fuel (glucose) but neither should particularly be banned from the candidiasis patient's diet. On the other hand if you only eat fruits and starches, you will rob your body of some very necessary amino acids which are used to rebuild and restore the immune system among other things. So a moderate diet is best with emphasis on vegetables and quality protein. We believe that eating or not eating any particular food will not cause or bring back candidiasis. If diet caused or cured candidiasis, it would not be the problem it is today.

STATEMENT: The Only Way To Treat Systemic Candidiasis Is With Nystatin And Nyzoral, Which Are Anti-Yeast/Anti-Fungal Drugs Commonly Used By Most Medical Doctors.

FACT: False. Let's first take a look at Nystatin. This is an effective drug for gut candidiasis but it is effective because it is so poorly absorbed that it remains in the intestinal tract and does a great job of killing yeast. The temporary feeling of improvement that the individual who has Systemic Candidiasis experiences is due to the loss of the toxic load from the overgrowth in the gut, not from any removal or destruction of the yeast infestation internally.

Nyzoral is a trade name for Ketoconazole, a drug which is very highly toxic to the liver, has the most emphatic warning given to a drug in the Physician's Desk Reference as to its toxicity. It is effective internally but you run the risk of irreversible damage to your liver or even a fatal reaction from this drug.

STATEMENT: <u>Candidiasis Can Be Sexually Transmitted.</u>

FACT: <u>True.</u> The sexual act can transmit the yeast to either partner. In the male it is not as likely such transmission will result in Systemic Candidiasis, but it can create a chronic source of reinfection of the female who may have been able to free herself of contamination with one treatment or another.

STATEMENT: <u>The Use Of Pau D'Arco Tea, Garlic, And Caprylic Acid Will Control Systemic Candidiasis.</u>

FACT: <u>Partially True.</u> These substances do have

anti-yeast/anti-fungal properties but like Nystatin are far more effective in the gut than they are internally. The benefit may not be complete enough to say that the yeast is out of the body. Both garlic and caprylic acid are good fungicides and can be of benefit. We just have not found them effective alone.

STATEMENT: The Oral Use Of Special Strains Of Bacteria Which Produce Hydrogen Peroxide Will Control Systemic Candidiasis.

FACT: Less Than Partially True. Although hydrogen peroxide will destroy the yeast/fungus, remember that what these special strains of bacteria (acidophilus, etc) are trying to do is to repopulate the bacteria lost in the gut due to overdoses of antibiotics. They do not normally migrate internally thus they will not reduce systemic candidiasis infestations.

STATEMENT: There Is No Absolute Way To Determine If You Have Systemic Candidiasis Or Not.

FACT: True. Candidiasis is normal in the gut so a stool sample may only give you an idea that there is an overgrowth in the gut. The reaction-type studies indicate whether your body is sensitive to the yeast but can be very positive in individuals with no symptoms and marginally positive or even negative on individuals who are loaded with symptoms. Blood tests indicate the amount of antibodies present which means that you have been fighting or are fighting yeast, but they do not differentiate between the two. The biggest misinformation they give is to the patient who has been treated and their symptoms are becoming less but the blood test will be positive. The very best test, in our opinion, is whether or not you have the symptoms on the Candida Questionnaire which follows at the end of this section - and whether or not these symptoms can be traced to any other problem.

WHOLISTIC THERAPY
(As practiced at Hospital Santa Monica, Institut Santa Monica and The Al - Don Institute)

Most physicians and health practitioners who have seen a reasonable number of candidiasis patients well know the frustration which often develops as you try to help the patient recover from symptoms which often are vague and of the type that are usually associated with hypochondria or mental illness.

We have formerly mentioned the many products touted in the "health periodicals" as home remedies and which are often of some benefit. But it was not until we began using oxygen therapy, more specifically in the form of intravenous hydrogen peroxide, oral hydrogen and magnesium peroxides and rectal ozone that we began to see predictable results.

Intravenous infusion of hydrogen peroxide has proven to be one of the most dramatic healing agents I have ever witnessed. By increasing the oxygen content in both the venous and arterial blood, miraculous things happen. Specifically for Systemic Candidiasis patients, you find allergies disappearing in five to ten days and a clearance of the yeast from the interior of the body within 10 infusions or less. To the chronic sufferer this sounds absolutely unbelievable because there is no other treatment available that will produce such results in such a short period of time. Our records indicate that these are reasonable statements.

PEROXIDE - OZONE - OXYGEN

We should examine hydrogen peroxide, magnesium peroxide, ozone and other forms of liquid oxygen to determine what it is they have to offer. First we must understand that all of these items have only one thing to offer the body when they are broken down - oxygen. And we must appreciate that oxygen has two major functions:

    1. Oxygen is one of the two major ingredients necessary to create energy. Oxygen loss creates problems for every organ, tissue and cell of the body because without energy they cannot do their job. This energy loss is also one of the most significant problems we face in the Systemic Candidiasis or Chronic Fatigue Syndrome patient.

2. Oxygen is the greatest detoxifier that the body knows. By initiating the oxidation reduction system within the body, oxygen sets forth the pathway in which potentially very toxic metabolic waste can be altered into a tolerable waste product that can be more easily eliminated through normal excretion channels. This occurs by the simple combining of oxygen with the toxic material.

When oxygen is deficient, most of the oxygen which is present will be used in the energy-producing-mechanism since this is the most critical for life. Thus we can see that the very symptoms so prevalent in both Systemic Candidiasis and Chronic Fatigue Syndrome - loss of energy and toxic symptoms such as allergies - are directly related to the oxygen content of the body.

There are several ways in which we can increase the oxygen content of the body. Here are some of the more simple ways:

1. Deep Breathing - If someone is asked to take a deep breath, they inevitably will suck in their lower abdomen and lift their shoulders while inhaling. This is exactly the wrong way to breathe deeply! If you have ever watched a baby breathe, you will see the lower abdomen move up and down with each breath. They automatically know that the best way to utilize the full capacity of the lung is to breathe down

and not up. It seems as we get older we somehow lose that innate knowledge and primarily only use the upper part of the lungs in a very shallow manner. Voice and wind instrument teachers always teach diaphragmatic breathing which uses that powerful muscle to assist in totally filling the lungs. It would behoove you to spend five minutes two or three times daily to concentrate on breathing down, down, down and not lifting your shoulders when you breathe deeply. One way to do this very easily, and a position in which it is impossible to not breathe deeply, is the following: Lie flat on your back facing a sofa. Lift your legs up and move your hips against the sofa, now rest your legs from the knees down on the sofa. Breathing in this position guarantees you will get the most possible use out of your lungs.

2. Exercise - Some form of exercise which will raise your heart rate to 120 beats per minute or more will produce deep breathing automatically. Rapid walking is the safest from a body viewpoint, resulting in less injuries than any other form, but the use of a mini-trampoline, a stepper, a stationary bicycle or a treadmill are all excellent.

But when you are ill and not feeling well, more dramatic and intensive efforts may be necessary. You can increase your oxygen level by the use of liquid products which are exceptionally high in bound oxygen. Hydrogen peroxide is one of them. Magnesium peroxide is another, chlorine peroxide is another. Ozone is a powerful oxygen donor and has been utilized for years on the European Continent for all manner of diseases. Up until very recently, ozone was so unstable that it could not be locked in a stable liquid solution. However, recently we were able to accomplish this and have liquid ozone solutions that do not release their oxygen for several months or until activated by the saliva in the mouth.

Liquid ozone is fairly tasteless and is well tolerated. But hydrogen peroxide is really obnoxious, particularly in any concentration high enough to gain benefit. Several years ago Dr. Donsbach found a way to alter 35% food-grade hydrogen peroxide so that the metallic aftertaste was almost totally eliminated. This has permitted individuals who are interested in using this product to regularly consume it without discomfort. Hydrogen peroxide is the least expensive of all the liquid oxygen products, but the ozone is easier to use for some. Again it must be emphasized that the only thing we are after is the oxygen so you can choose your own method. At the present time, research has found that magnesium peroxide is also an effective method of obtaining oxygen through oral ingestion.

Hydrogen peroxide can also be infused directly into the blood stream through an intravenous feeding.

Some doctors have now tried this method and are using it, but they are few and far between. It is by no means an accepted or endorsed procedure by the medical profession officials. In fact they condemn it and periodically plant horror stories in the press to discourage people from taking advantage of this simple and safe remedy.

Ozone can be administered in a variety of ways, but the method which we have found to be the most effective and practical is by rectal insufflation. Here, a soft rubber catheter is inserted into the rectum and medical grade ozone is released in quantities of from one-half to one full liter. The patient is encouraged to retain this as long as possible and the effect of this form of delivery have been found to be greater than any other form. It can be used every day or even twice a day in those serious cases which require it.

In those facilities which we have control of, the oxygen therapies are administered as follows:
  1. From 3 to 8 fluid ounces of a liquid mixture containing hydrogen and magnesium peroxides with each ounce containing the equivalent oxygen as you would find in 20 drops of pure 35% hydrogen peroxide.
  2. 10 infusions of hydrogen peroxide containing the 35% hydrogen peroxide and DMSO.
  3. Daily rectal insufflations of ozone.

OTHER THERAPY

It should be obvious that we find many other therapies necessary to overcome the many symptoms of Systemic Candidiasis and Chronic Fatigue Syndrome. The adrenals play a large part in the recovery of these patients. Anyone who has worked with these conditions can usually find both objective and subjective signs of adrenal exhaustion.

We are fortunate in Mexico to still have access to adrenal cortex extract (ACE) which has historically been one of the most effective medicines known to assist in rehabilitating the adrenal glands. We use it as a nasal spray, since our knowledge of the absorptive ability of the nasal mucosa has certainly been enhanced by the efficiency of the use of illicit, unnecessary drugs through this means. It is simple for the patient and dosage can easily be controlled. No more need for injections to get the benefits desired.

Several nutrients are particularly important for adrenal rehabilitation and we use considerable pantothenic acid, vitamin C and potassium as well as homeopathic concentrates of adrenal tissue.

Another substance we use is isoprinosine, an antiviral, which is possibly one of the best immune stimulants known to man today. Here we have another substance which is not available in the U.S. but is commonly used throughout the world. It is an effective and safe medicine for use in this way.

We are very interested in the thymus gland since it is the seat or center of the immune system. You will read more about this later, but do be aware that the constant irritation of the immune system by either of the organisms associated with Candidiasis or Chronic Fatigue Syndrome is almost sure to create serious problems with the thymus. Lack of attention to this will leave the patient half well (if such is possible).

SPECIAL DIET

The use of a special candida or chronic fatigue syndrome diet is NOT part of our protocol. Patients are all fed a wholesome and varied diet with encouragement to sparingly consume those foods which they were formerly allergic. Our basic diet consists of the following guidelines:

    1. Consume at least 1 bowlful of whole grain cereal every morning. This can be oatmeal or any other single or mixed grains, hot or cold as you wish.

    2. Consume at least 4 cupfuls of vegetables daily - cooked or raw.

    3. Consume at least one cupful of fresh fruit daily.

    4. Avoid all forms of concentrated sugars incl-

uding fruit juice. Eat the whole fruit!

4. Use only butter, olive oil and peanut oil as fats in your cooking. NO HYDROGENATED OILS OF ANY KIND ARE TO BE USED!

5. If you must, allow yourself one "sin" day per week to indulge your junk food cravings. Set the day and do not deviate or cheat. You will soon find out that as you eliminate the daily intake of these "food-less" foods, they lose their desirability.

6. As you wish or your principles allow, fish, cheese, eggs, quality meats, etc. can be consumed as your needs dictate. It should be obvious if you follow the dictates of the first three rules, there will not be enough room to overindulge in these foods. They are excellent sources of nutrients for man, but have had too much emphasis at the expense of the all important vegetables in our diet.

REGARDING ACIDOPHILUS

The average patient may wish to reimplant some friendly bacteria in the intestinal tract. Eating yogurt type foods will help with this but if you wish to aggressively reimplant the bacteria, here are the suggestions we give:

1. Use 5 capsules of a 1 billion live bacteria per capsule product at 11 a.m. and 5 capsules at 5 p.m. for a period of ten days.

2. Wait twenty days and repeat.

3. If you feel the second implantation has not been successful, you may wish to dissolve from five to ten capsules in about one pint of warm water and use it as a retention enema.

It is important that you take acidophilus capsules on an empty stomach - at least 45 minutes before a meal or three hours after a meal - for them to be effective. Contrary to what some believe, these capsules are not effective if taken with food in the stomach.

PROTECTION AGAINST REINFECTION

Candidiasis can be transmitted sexually so both partners should be aware of what can be done to prevent transferance during the sexual act.

MEN - Buy regular 3% hydrogen peroxide in the store and wash the genital area with this before and after intercourse. Just to be on the safe side do it a minimum of once a week.

WOMEN - A douche containing hydrogen peroxide is available which prevents contamination in the vaginal area. Also boric acid vaginal suppositories which are excellent yeast and fungal destroyers can be procured. Either one or a combination of both of these as a preventive or treatment for simple vaginal infections makes a lot of sense.

Once you have cleared your body of these invaders

keeping them out is not too much of a problem. We must constantly be aware of avoiding steroid containing drugs and antibiotics which can again predispose the body to infestation.

CANDIDIASIS & THE IMMUNE SYSTEM

At the very beginning of this booklet we talked about which came first - the chicken or the egg. This same dilemma faces us when we investigate the relationship between the immune system and the disorder we call Systemic Candidiasis.

There is no question in anyone's mind that the presence of Systemic Candidiasis can stress the immune system and over a period of time cause it to become so overworked it becomes unable to resist the entry of unwanted invaders.

The other side of this question is that the entry of the candida organism into the body is certainly made easier if the immune system is already tired and worn out. This phenomenon is often seen in the critically ill when candidiasis makes a strong entry in many parts of the body after the patient becomes ill. We must constantly be aware that organisms of all kinds are always on the ready to take up residence in our body and the presence of a vigilant immune system is the only force that keeps them out.

Most of us in the healing profession have wondered at one time or another why the immune system seems to be incapacitated for apparently no reason in some individuals. Such debilitation cannot be traced to an unhealthy life style or any chronic infection or infestation such as candidiasis. Now and then we find an infected root canal or the presence of active amalgam (mercury) leaking from a filled tooth. But frankly, most of the time we are in a quandry to explain why the immune system is not functioning.

Both of the authors have used darkfield microscopy for some time to observe the blood, but a recent discovery by Dr. Alsleben has opened a whole new vista in how we look at a slide. His observance and correlation of what we had always dismissed as "something" in the darkfield as we looked at it, may be the beginning of our understanding why the immune system is depleted for no apparent reason.

The "something" referred to is the presence of tiny, extremely active dots on the microscopic field. It is amazing how many have seen these organisms and never questioned what they were. Most of the time the observer is so interested in looking at what he knows is there that the eye probably doesn't even register what is present but unknown.

Dr. Alsleben used an unusual, advanced technique to observe these "dots" and concluded that they were the most highly active organism he had ever observed and further that they seemed to obtain their energy from the larger components of the blood stream. This follows a law of physics which says that energy will flow from a body of lesser energy to a body of greater energy. A properly focused darkfield microscope will allow you to observe these frantic microbes going to parts of the immune system such as the white cells and momentarily stop, then darting off.

The stop is apparently for the purpose of refueling, which depletes the cell of the energy stolen from it. When we observe individuals who are very sick, it is a guaranteed fact that we will find swarms of these active microbes which we have named "Kleptic Microbes" because they are constantly stealing energy from the other elements in the blood.

This phenomenon would be the same if you were lying in a pool of water infested with leeches. Although one leech could hardly take enough blood from you to cause any problem, if there were thousands of them draining your life blood away, you would soon become weak and unable to move.

The same appears to be the fact in the case of the immune system. Drawing liberally upon the wisdom of others and combining our own experience, the authors have devised a concoction of substances which will rapidly deplete the blood stream of these "Kleptic Microbes" and allow the rejuvenation of the immune system to progress in an orderly and rapid fashion.

Our patients are amazed to see the difference between the darkfield microscopic appearance of their blood after just one or two infusions of this mixture. This discovery has enabled us to give an educated and honest answer to the patient who says "Why can't I get rid of this feeling of utter, complete fatigue that I have?"

Most of these patients have been to countless doctors and have had a variety of approaches to their problem. Usually they have responded partially to some of the therapies but then they seem to revert right back to where they were. Our answer is that the candida organism was probably temporarily controlled by the method the doctor was using but the Kleptic Microbe was still there to keep the immune system down. So the first opportunity that candida, or whatever other organism was present, had to come back, it faced no defense system to prevent its return.

It is interesting to note that we see far more Kleptic Microbes in the blood of the Chronic Fatigue Syndrome patient than we do of the Systemic Candidiasis patient. This is probably why the CFS patient actually hurts more and has more sore throats, swollen lymph glands and other symptoms.

SYSTEMIC CANDIDIASIS
AND
CHRONIC FATIGUE SYNDROME

There is some confusion in the minds of some as to the difference between candidiasis and chronic fatigue syndrome. Candidiasis is associated with a yeast organism while chronic fatigue syndrome is associated with the Epstein Barr Virus. These authors are not too sure that it makes much difference which you have and the puzzling thing is that many of our patients have evidence of both. Looking at it in that light, we might just consider that the wholistic treatment we propose would effectively treat either or both as well as a host of other conditions which your body might be suffering from.

An official look at the Chronic Fatigue Syndrome says that it "may be nothing more than a wastebasket of diagnostic confusion." Other "experts," particularly those in Europe, would like to call it "Fibromyalgia" because it exhibits the symptoms of that disease: fatigue, myalgias (muscle pain) and sleep disturbances. In Great Britain, they tend to refer to it as "ME,' a contracture form of myalgic encephalomyelitis. This is characterized by both fatigue and emotional depression. An inability to release lactic acid from the muscle seems to explain the muscle fatigue, no explanation is offered for the depression. All these different names has led to confusion and an attempt was made to set up a criteria, or set of symptoms, that could be indicative of the elusive "Chronic Fatigue Syndrome." We print it here because it has the blessing of the foremost health epidemiologists and clinicians studying this disease.

A case of the chronic fatigue syndrome must fulfill major criteria 1 and 2, and the following minor criteria: six or more of the 11 symptom criteria and two or more of the three physical criteria, or eight or more of the 11 symptom criteria.

Major Criteria

1. New onset of persistent or relapsing, debilitating fatigue or easy fatigability in a person who has no previous history of similar symptoms, that does not resolve with bed rest and that is severe enough to reduce or impair average daily activity below 50% of the patient's premorbid activity level for a period of at least six months.

2. Other clinical conditions that may produce similar symptoms must be excluded by thorough evaluation based on history, physical examination, and appropriate laboratory findings. These conditions include:

malignancy - autoimmune disease - localized infection - chronic or subacute bacterial disease - fungal disease - parasitic disease - HIV infection - chronic psychiatric disease - hysterical personality disorder- anxiety - schizophrenia - neuromuscular disorder-chronic use of tranquilizers or anti-depressant medication - chronic inflammatory disease - endocrine disease - drug dependency or abuse - side effects of a chronic medication or other toxic agent - chronic pulmonary, cardiac, gastrointestinal, hepatic or hematologic disease.

Minor Criteria

To fulfill a symptom criteria, a symptom must have begun at or after the time of onset of increased fatigability and must have persisted or recurred over a period of at least six months (individual symptoms may or may not have occurred simultaneously).

Symptom Criteria

1. Mild fever - oral temperature between 37.5 C (99.5 F) and 38.6 C (101.5 F)   Note: oral temperatures over 38.6 C should prompt studies for other causes of illness.

2. Sore throat.

3. Painful lymph nodes in the anterior or posterior cervical or axillary distribution.

4. Unexplained generalized muscle weakness.

5. Muscle discomfort or myalgia.

6. Prolonged generalized fatigue after levels of exercise that would have been easily tolerated in the patient's premorbid state.

7. Generalized headaches of a different type than may have occurred prior to onset.

8. Migratory arthralgia without joint swelling or redness.

9. Neuropsychologic complaints (one or more of the following: photophobia, transient visual scotomata, forgetfulness, excessive irritiability, confusion, difficulty thinking, inability to concentrate, depression).

10. Sleep disturbance (hypersomnia or insomnia).

11. Description of the main symptom complex as initially developing over a few hours to a few days (this is not a true symptom, but may be considered as equivalent to the above symptoms in meeting the requirements of the case definition).

Physical Criteria

Physical criteria must be documented by a physician on at least two occasions, at least one month apart.

1. Low grade fever - oral temperature between 37.6 C and 38.6 C, or rectal temperature between 37.8 C and 38.8 C.

2. Nonexudative pharyngitis.

3. Palpable or tender anterior or posterior cervical or axillary lymph nodes.

Although the criteria considered many physiological factors, social and psychological factors such as overwork, chronic stress and drug or alcohol abuse should be excluded. Anemias should be excluded but vitamin and mineral deficiencies should be considered.

* * *

There you have the thoughts and feelings of some of the most respected physicians in their fields. These thoughts to come to mind:

1. Under the physical symptoms the doctor must wait at least 31 days before he treats either a low grade fever, a sore throat or enlarged lymph nodes. What patient is going to wait that long if they have those symptoms? You'll find another doctor!

2. Another criteria is that the symptom must have persisted or recurred over a perod of at least six months. This seems ridiculous because the average physician will not treat without a diagnosis and to make a patient wait for six months is unreasonable.

It would appear that these criteria are designed to never allow a physician to make the diagnosis of Chronic Fatigue Syndrome. And from the patients we see on a daily basis, this is just about what is happening. The diagnosis comes from the knowledge the patient has or has obtained from friends. This unwillingness on the part of physicians to accept a new diagnosis of a disease which is different from anything they have seen is unfortunate.

We see many patients who have chased the elusive "Epstein Barr Virus" as a progenitor of the Chronic Fatigue Syndrome. Because we have seen many patients who tested positive for the EBV titer who were quite sick and others equally high who had no symptoms at all, we are convinced that it is the state of the immune system that determines which person will develop the symptoms of Chronic Fatigue Syndrome and who will not.

This actually makes our job easier, allowing us to concentrate much of our therapy on those things we know about - such as the Kleptic Microbe - which deprive us of the immunity we need to oppose disease of all kinds. The Kleptic Microbe Immune Modulator Vaccine has been a real help to us in preventing recurrences of these type of problems.

CANDIDA - AIDS CONNECTION

It will be very important for us to understand the definition of AIDS in order to achieve a proper perspective of the relationship between AIDS and Candidiasis. This will be vital in determining the AIDS risk for a person infected with Candida Yeast.

Here is a published definition of AIDS:

"AIDS is best known for producing an inability of the body's immune system to ward off infections. It is known that a person acquires the full-blown disease or its precursor conditions by becoming infected with the AIDS virus. The most highly-publicized aspect of the AIDS virus is its penchant for attacking and disabling the white blood cells which normally ward off infection. These white blood cells, called Helper T-cells, normally serve to activate other cells which produce antibodies that attack invading organisms.

When the AIDS virus invades these white blood cells, their ability to defend against infection is seriously impaired. The Helper T-cells lose their normal role and become AIDS virus factories. In the process, the T-cells are gradually destroyed, and as they disappear the main initiator of the immune system is lost. This effectively devastates the immune system." (G. Antonio - THE AIDS COVERUP)

What we all must now realize is that the AIDS retro-lenti virus kills an individual by destroying the immune system which causes the individual to be destroyed by primary and secondary infections against which it cannot defend itself.

A disorder associated with AIDS so frequently that it characterizes the AIDS victim is fungus infection. The most common of all fungal infections is Candidiasis. What may not have been fully appreciated is the relationship between fungal infections and AIDS.

"The weaker a person's immune system becomes, by whatever cause, the more inviting a target it becomes for other infections. The more it is attacked by new germs, the weaker it becomes. In the terminal stages of AIDS, patients are victimized by unrelenting, multiple infections. People who die of AIDS actually die of the complications of unopposed infection caused by the assemblage of germs."
(Slaff - THE AIDS EPIDEMIC)

AIDS weakens the immune system but so does candidiasis. And so does the Kleptic Microbe. Which comes first? Is it possible to actually repel the AIDS virus if we have a strong immune system not overrun with Kleptic Microbes and candida organisms? We don't have a solid answer to that question, but it certainly bears some serious consideration.

One of the first medical publications on the subject of AIDS indicated a principal reason for the concentration of AIDS in homosexual men. It was that their sexual habits included anal intercourse. This was based upon the theory that anal intercourse might deposit sperm in the vicinity of bleeding blood vessels enabling the sperm to get into the blood stream and cause a profound shock to the immune system. If sperm can be absorbed through an open vessel in membranes such as found in the rectal area, can such materials be absorbed through the membranes of other structures like the vagina, mouth or lungs?

A description of the sperm cell will be helpful in this understanding. A sperm cell consists of a head and a tail. The head contains genetic nuclear material and possibly viruses and bacteria. It has been known for more than fifteen years that the degenerating sperm within an individual, such as one who has had a vasectomy, can produce or cause autoimmune reactions within the individual that can best be described as neurological disorders such as multiple sclerosis.

Thus the deposition of sperm into the rectal area can create a cascade of immune problems that make rectal intercourse under any circumstances a practice to be seriously considered before indulging in. Another less known fact is that the vaginal tract in the female can be less protective than is thought.

"The association of sperm-induced immune dysregulation with the practice of anal intercourse underscores the critical structural differences between the rectum and the vagina. While the lining of the vaginal mucosa comprises a squamous multilayer epithelium capable of protecting against any abrasive effect during intercourse, the lining of the rectum is a single layer of columnar epithelium." Mavligit - SUPPORT FOR THE HYPOTHESIS THAT SPERMATOZOA INDUCE IMMUNE DYSREGULATION IN HOMOSEXUAL MALES - JAMA

This article would lead one to believe that there is almost perfect protection in vaginal intercourse. This is simply not true. While it is true that the female who has a normal level of estrogen will maintain a multi-layered vaginal wall, how about the multitude of females who are deficient in estrogen, who have had hysterectomies, etc?

There is a test that any concerned female should take. It is unfortunate that it is not more common because it could prevent the unknowing transmission of viruses and other bacteria through the vaginal wall. The test is called a Cytogram Maturation Index. It determines how much of the vaginal wall has been lost due to structural weakening as a result of deficient female hormones. Many women, even the young, may have lost a great deal of their vaginal tissue. This is the reason for easy abrasion, dryness and frequent infections in the so-called "menopausal" vaginas.

Knowing that the vaginal wall is not a perfect barrier to alien life form leads us directly to the fact that the vaginal wall may be an entry port for life forms such as:

| bacteria | parasites | fungus |
| viruses | yeast | protozoa |

Many times the common yeast infection of the vaginal tract is treated locally and although the yeast may be temporarily destroyed in the area, were any preventive measures taken to insure that the local infection did not travel through the wall and into the systemic circulation?

This route of infection might be more prevalent than we would like to admit and would provide for a constant immune system stress which might lead to immune system deficiency which might lead to an easy road for other infections, particularly those of a viral nature to become virulent.

THERAPY SIDE-EFFECTS

There have been complaints from patients that they become quite sick during therapy and feel or have been told this is due to "die-off." Let's take a look at what happens when an agent is used that partially disintegrates the cell wall of a yeast organism. Once the yeast cell is ruptured, the inner contents can escape and readily pass through the absorptive membrane of the intestinal wall causing a low-level immune challenge and a detoxification crisis.

This certainly is a cause for concern. Are these anti-yeast, anti-fungal drugs actually creating their own new problems that may predispose the patient to new symptoms? Is this why the great majority of patients treated with these drugs have a temporary feeling that they are getting better and then soon relapse into the same problems they had before?

We believe this is the case and propose the treatment protocol that we use for the Systemic Candidiasis and Chronic Fatigue Syndrome patient does not result in the "die-off" syndrome because of the heavy emphasis we place on oxygen therapy. Because oxygen is the great detoxifier, there is no overage of waste product when the organism is destroyed and our patients do not usually have any of the symptoms described before.

SUMMARY

Systemic Candidiasis and Chronic Fatigue Syndrome are real problems in our society today. They are becoming of epidemic proportions but the average physician is finding it difficult to make these diagnosis, because it is believed they are "trend" diseases and really exist mostly in the minds of the patient.

Because of this attitude many individuals are suffering needlessly. Some are relegated to the psychiatric maze which is often difficult to escape and others become outcasts, even within their own family. We feel there is a logical and proper way to approach this problem and offer this booklet as our answer to the multitudes who are seeking relief.

There is no panacea for any disorder of the body but a careful evaluation will usually find the keys which allow a physician to slowly and surely remove the causes which created the condition. Removal of the Kleptic Microbe allows proper rebuilding of the immune system. Destruction of the organism - be it yeast or virus - is only a matter of time and proper application of known principles.

By not introducing toxic drugs, by removing causes and restoring function, health must inevitably result.

CANDIDA TESTS

There are many tests for the candida organism. It is easy to elucidate in either the stool or in vaginal secretions. Such testing has litttle, if any, bearing on systemic candidiasis.

Blood tests are not terribly relevant since the yeast does not take up residence in the blood but instead prefers to find moist, mucus membranes such as in the lungs and sinuses.

Skin reaction tests will demonstrate the presence of antibodies but are not good indicators as to whether or not you are overwhelmed with Systemic Candidiasis.

Therfore the test on the following pages is as good a test as we know for screening yourself. As with all tests, it is not infallable but it does give a strong indication of some problem that needs attention. Take the time to answer all the questions and determine what your possible susceptibility to this unwanted intruder is.

CANDIDIASIS QUESTIONNAIRE
AND SCORE SHEET

This questionnaire is designed for adults and the scoring system isn't appropriate for children. It lists factors in your medical history which promote the growth of candida albicans (Section A), and symptoms commonly found in individuals with yeast-connected illness (Section B and C).

For each "Yes" answer in Section A, circle the Point Score in that section. Total your score and record it in the box at the end of the section. Then move on to Sections B and C and score as directed.

Filling out and scoring this questionnaire should help you and your physician evaluate the possible role of candida in contributing to your health problems. Yet it will not provide an automatic "Yes" or "No" answer.

Section A: History

1. Have you taken tetracyclines
(Sumycin, Panmycin, Vibramycin, Minocin,
etc.) or other antibiotics for acne for 1 month
or more?   35

2. Have you, at any time in your life
taken other "broad spectrum" antibiotics for
respiratory, urinary or other infections (for 2
months or longer, or in shorter courses 4 or
more times in a 1-year period?)   35

3. Have you taken a broad spectrum
antibiotic drug - even a single course?   ·   6

4. Have you, at any time in your life,
been bothered by persistent prostatitis, vagin-
itis or other problems affecting your repro-
ductive organs?   25

5. Have been pregnant 2 or more times.   5
      1 time.   3

6. Have taken birth control pills for more
than 2 years.   15
      For 6 months to 2 years.   8

7. Have you taken prednisone, Dec-
dron or other cortisone-type drugs...
     For more than 2 weeks?   15
     For 2 weeks or less?   6

8. Does exposure to perfumes, insect-
icides, fabric shop odors and other chemicals
     Provoke moderate to severe symptoms?   20
     Mild symptoms?   5

9. Are your symptoms worse on damp,
muggy days or in moldy places?   20

10. Have you had athlete's foot, ring
worm, "jock itch" or other chronic fungus infections of the skin or nails? Have these been
     Severe or persistent?   20
     Mold to moderate?   10

11. Do you crave sugar?   10

12. Do you crave bread?   10

13. Do you crave alcohol?   10

14. Does tobacco smoke bother you?   10

Total Score, Section A _____

SECTION B: MAJOR SYMPTOMS

For each of your symptoms, enter the appropriate figure in the Point Score Column:

If a symptom is occasional or mild............3 points
If a symptom is frequent or moderate.......6 points
If a symptom is severe or disabling............9 points

Add total score and record it in the box at the end of this section.

score

1. Fatigue or lethargy _____
2. Feeling of being "drained" _____
3. Poor memory _____
4. Feeling of "spaciness" _____
5. Depression _____
6. Numbness, burning, tingling _____
7. Muscle aches _____
8. Muscle weakness _____
9. Pain, swelling in joints _____
10. Abdominal pain _____
11. Constipation _____
12. Diarrhea _____
13. Bloating _____
14. Vaginal discharge _____
15. Vaginal burning or itching _____
16. Prostatitis _____
17. Impotence _____
18. Loss of sexual desire _____
19. Endometriosis _____

20. Menstrual cramps   _____

21. Premenstrual tension   _____

22. Spots in front of eyes   _____

23. Erratic vision   _____

Total Score......................_____

SECTION C: OTHER SYMPTOMS

For each of your symptoms enter the appropriate figure in the score column:

If a symptom is occasional or mild..............1 point

If a symptom is frequent or moderate.........2 points

If a symptom is frequent or disabling.........3 points

Add total score and record it in the box at the end of the section.

             score

1. Drowsiness   _____

2. Irritability or jitteriness   _____

3. Incoordination   _____

4. Inability to concentrate   _____

5. Frequent mood swings   _____

6. Headache   _____

7. Dizziness/loss of balance _____

8. Ear pressure   _____

9. Head swelling   _____

10. Itching   _____

11. Other rashes   _____

12. Heartburn   _____

13. Indigestion   _____

14. Belching and burping _____
15. Flatulence _____
16. Mucus in stool _____
17. Hemorrhoids _____
18. Dry mouth _____
19. Rash/blisters in mouth _____
20. Bad breath _____
21. Joint swelling or arthritis _____
22. Nasal congestion or discharge _____
23. Postnasal drip _____
24. Nasal itching _____
25. Sore or dry throat _____
26. Cough _____
27. Itching ears _____
28. Wheezing or shortness of breath _____
29. Urgency or urinary frequency _____
30. Burning on urination _____
31. Failing vision _____
32. Burning or tearing of eyes _____
33. Recurrent infections of ears _____
34. Ear pain _____

Total Score......................_____

Total Score, Section A _____

Total Score, Section B _____

Total Score, Section C _____

GRAND TOTAL _____

Evaluation

The Grand Total Score will help you and your practitioner of the healing arts determine if your health problems are yeast-connected. Scores in women will run higher as 7 items in the questionnaire apply exclusively to women, while only 2 apply exclusively to men.

Women   **Over 180**
Men   **Over 140**
Yeast-connected health problems are almost certainly present.

Women   **Over 120**
Men   **Over 90**
Yeast-connected health problems are probably present in these cases.

Women   **Over 60**
Men   **Over 40**
Yeast-connected health problems are possibly present in these cases.

Women   **Less than   60**
Men   **Less than   40**
Yeast is probably not involved in any health problems.

AN EPIDEMIC

There are an increasing number of physicians and clinics that are attempting to treat the Systemic Candidiasis problem so we sent for their literature. The descriptions of the therapies that were being used and the reported degree of effectiveness did not match up with the reports that our patients gave us.

In interviewing patients who had been under antifungal therapy or who had completed therapy in other centers around the country, we found the following:

1. About half of the patients treated by the clinics surveyed reported that they felt better initially and then began to regress to a state that was not as good as when they had started their programs. The therapies that were used on these patients were essentially oral anti-fungal antibiotic medications and a carbohydrate restrictive diet.

2. The concensus of our patient surveys indicated that the method of therapy just described was not very effective. The probable explanation was that the therapy was not directed to the cause of the patient's complex disorder.

Thus the accepted method of treatment in the "candida clinics" was really not effective.

The most scary facet of this condition is the large number of individuals who are totally unaware of what they have and what can be done about it. Careful questioning of patients about their signs and symptoms have led us to an alarming number of positive diagnosis in patients who were concerned about their health problems but had no clue as to its possible orgin.

This can have far-reaching effects since whatever allowed the infestation to occur may continue to smolder until the difficulty is severe enough to create serious problems that could have easily been averted with early confrontation. By the time this happens your general state of health and the integrity of your immune system may be disturbed to the point of allowing a low-level chronic infection to exist which allows other "opportunistic" infections to flourish.

This becomes especially true for those infected with the AIDS virus. Such debility of the immune system can soon be followed by serious illness and death.

When you become aware of the principal symptoms of this disease process, a great many will come to the realization that you are probably infested with the condition of Candida yeast infection. The information presented in this booklet can then help you make up your mind as to what you wish to do about it.

THE KLEPTIC MICROBE

Let's take another look at the Kleptic Microbe, a tiny, highly-energetic dot on a high resolution darkfield microscopic examination. We are sure that we did not discover this microbe. In fact we are quite sure that it has been discovered several times in the past century and promptly relegated to the scrap pile of medical non-interest.

In 1934, Doctor von Brehmer isolated a specific organism from human blood which he called the *Siphon-Spora Polymorpha*. He believed that this organism could well be the basic cause of all illness.

In later years of research, von Brehmer found that if the pH level of the blood became more alkaline, perhaps 7.45 or above, the organism became identifiable with tumor growth. He was able to culture the organism from many human tumors as well as the blood of the person with the tumors. The more that von Brehmer searched, the more places within the body could the organism be found.

He described the organism as being highly **pleomorphic** (meaning capable of changing shape and form to accomodate the environment it is in) and capable of changing into mycelial (yeast) fungal forms, sporangia and spore forms.

We believe that the Kleptic Microbe that we observe in every case of serious disease that we see is the same *Siphon-Spora Polymorpha* that Doctor von Brehmer described. This highly mobile microbe is something to watch in the darkfield microscope. It darts to and fro going from one blood component to another, stealing energy from each as it momentarily stops. In serious cases we see swarms of these organisms clouding the microscopic field; in less serious disease states, we usually see less.

Dr. von Brehmer came to the conclusion that this microbe was not only associated with cancer but also several other diseases, including arthritis. We feel that we have confirmed this association as well as its presence in Systemic Candidiasis and Chronic Fatigue Syndrome. Its characteristic of "stealing" energy from other particles in the blood stream certainly fits in well with what we know about these conditions.

PARASITES

There is another very important abnormality that can occur in your bowel. To demonstrate this, here is a case of an industrious middle aged man with a wonderful family. He appeared to be in normal good health except he complained of chest pains and excessive fatigue. He had been examined by two very good doctors for possible heart or circulatory problems. These tests came out within normal limits so he was told it probably was the tension from his work.

This was reassuring to some extent except that the chest pains continued. They would occur with or without exertion and even during his sleep. The distribution of the pain was classic for coronary artery disease, yet the stress treadmill electrocardiogram was negative. He decided to try wholistic medicine and came to our hospital.

Infra-red Electronic Thermography revealed a tremendous instability of the superior cervical sympathetic ganglion and the posterior nerve roots of the first thoracic nerves. Why the nervous instability? There was no history of trauma and no apparent spinal abberation. His blood chemistries were even worse. He'd had his blood tested before, but our tests are far more comprehensive and provide information not available from routine blood tests on several body functions. The tests indicated a breakdown of vital muscle and other organ tissue. There was indication that his cells had increased their permeability and were leaking nutrients. There was an abundance of bacteria visible in his blood stream. There was one more abnormality. He had occult blood in his stools. This meant that his intestinal membrane was bleeding somewhere. It could have been cancer or perhaps small ulcerations had eroded through capillary blood vessels in the lining of the intestine.

If blood vessels were broken, open and hemorrhaging into the bowel lumen, would it be possible for microbes from the fecal content to get into the blood and into the lymphatic vessels? The answer would have to be - yes! Thus we demonstrate another way for yeast and other organisms to enter the blood stream and ravage the entire body. Another finding was present in this man's tests. A protozoal parasite was present. The organism is described thusly in a textbook:

"It is a pear -shaped organism half again as large as a red blood cell. It has a sucking disc under its front end. The organism has eight flagella whips that propel it through fluid. This organism lives high up in the intestinal tract and can cause significant inflammation of the intestinal wall.

These organisms can invade the mucosa and the absorptive layer of the intestinal wall, produce

63.

small ulcers and excrete hyaluronidase enzymes which aid in tissue destruction. The ulcers can become secondarily infected with intestinal bacteria. The entire bowel can become involved in the process and create a multitude of problems."

Once the organism is entrenched, there are five things that can happen:

1. The body completely destroys the organism.

2. The body will live in a peaceful coexistence, meaning that a chronic smouldering, damage producing infection will go on for years.

3. It will produce large ulcers.

4. It will pass through the capillary vessels, enter the protal circulation and lodge in the liver.

5. It will enter the general blood stream and infect the entire body.

We are happy to report that once proper anti-microbial treatment, along with our entire wholistic protocol was instituted, this gentleman again rejoined the land of the healthy. He was lucky in many respects that he had not been put on a lot of medications which might have masked some of the symptoms and allowed the condition to progress further. As it was, the full recovery period took six months because that many problems cannot be eradicated overnight. Almost all of his therapy was completed at home, except for his brief two week stay in the hospital. You might wonder why we present this case.

Simply because we find parasite infestation in many of our patients. This does not mean that parasites are their primary or only problem but it demonstrates how the other organisms can enter the body, how various factors may deplete the body energy in such a way that other opportunistic infections can attack us with a vengeance.

THE IMPORTANCE OF HCL

Hydrochloric acid is very important in the chain of events that lead to microbial infestation through the intestinal tract. The empty stomach of the "healthy individual" is usually free of microorganisms. Most all of the microbes that do reach this organ do so via saliva, nasopharyngeal secretions and food.

These organisms are usually killed by the high acidity and other digestive enzyme contents of the gastric juice. Those organisms that are not killed are passed into the intestines. In order to maintain the acid pH in the stomach capable of destroying these organisms, a person must be young and perfectly normal.

As an example an older person, 65 years of age for example, produces **eighty-five percent (85%) less hydrochloric acid than they did when they were twenty-five years of age.** An enormous number of people over the age of forty have serious deficiencies of hydrochloric acid in their stomachs. Think of the number of Americans who take antacid medicines every day to deliberately neutralize what they think are elevations of the stomach acids. How are these people going to destroy the incoming microbes?

One of the areas which we are very aware of is the state of the upper intestinal tract of our patient. They sometimes find it difficult to understand why we are so emphatic about the use of a broad spectrum digestive aid when they don't feel they have a digestive problem. However the majority of Systemic Candidiasis and Chronic Fatigue sufferers do have some digestive complaints.

A good digestive tablet or capsule will contain all of these ingredients:
>Betaine hydrochloride
>Pepsin
>Pancreatin
>Bile Salts
>Papain
>Bromelain

Dosage may vary from 2 to 5 tablets with each meal, depending upon severity of symptoms and size of meal. In general, individuals have less problems digesting starchy or carbohydrate-type foods than they do with protein and/or fat combinations. This does not mean the latter are less important, it only means they require more digestive effort.

WHERE DO THEY COME FROM ?

This part of this booklet is for those who would like to think a little, to speculate, to question. The question is: Where do germs and microbes and other creatures come from? Do they all have a "mommy and daddy?" Where are all the "baby" germs and microbes? Has anyone ever seen a germ give birth?

The reason we ask those questions is because we feel that in searching for answers to these questions, you might get some answers as to why modern medicine is going the wrong way in their treatment of disease. Their concept of disease "the Germ Theory" is wrong and we can prove it by their own science.

Many, many years ago, about 1675, an inquisitive scholar named Anton Leeuwenhoek had ground glass to make a crude microscope. In observing some rain water he had collected, he noted there were tiny organisms moving about in the water. He wondered where the "wee creatures" had come from. There were a variety of possibilities: they could have been in the ground that he had collected the rain water from, they could have been in the rain as it came down from the sky, or they could have been another of Gods creations that was just very tiny.

He determined that he would find out. Taking a clean

bowl, he set it out in the rain. When it had some rain in it, he rinsed the bowl with the rain water just to make sure and then collected some clean rain water. He put the water in several pipettes and then observed it under his special lenses.

The first thing he proved was that the rain water as it came from the sky did not contain the creatures, it was totally free of them. Hour after hour, day after day, he squinted at the rain water. On the fourth day he was rewarded - the "wee beasties" began to appear in the water.

He reported this to the circle of educated people that were to become the founders of the sciences as we know them today. One of them was the founder of chemistry as we know it, Robert Boyle; another was Sir Isaac Newton who wrote many of the principles of physics. This was also a time when religion played a big part in every major decision that was made.

The problem facing these scholars could be worded this way:

     1. The microbes were not in the rain water but later developed from nothing.

     2. The microbes were not in the rain water but later developed from something.

     3. The microbes were not in the rain water but flew or crept into the pipette from somewhere.

The theologians were quick to assert that it could not possibly be number one; something could not come from nothing. The scientists were quite convinced that the microbes came from somewhere else and thus they chose number three.

When Leeuwenhoek protested that the pippettes were sealed, they ignored him.

This self-styled scientific community strongly advocated the concept that every organism has a father-mother progenitor somewhere, thus the microbes could not have developed out of "something." Since the "mother-father" could not be located in the rain water, the microbes had to come from the air that was introduced whenever the water was exposed.

AND THUS WAS BORN THE GERM THEORY!

During the late eighteen hundreds, Doctor Pouchet sought to test the accuracy of the air germ theory. He passed hundreds of cubic meters of air through rain water and was never able to see the "wee beasties" until after the water had sat for four days.

He invented an apparatus that collected dust particles from the air and deposited them on glass plates. Pouchet then analyzed the dust. He conducted these experiments on glaciers in the Pyrenees, in the catacombs at Thebes and atop the cathedral in Rouen. He found many things, but only rarely did he find a "Wee Beastie" (they now had other names).

AND LIFE BEGINS

Here is a simple demonstration of a scientfic experiment that may make things clearer. It may also astound and confuse you.

Place a small amount of pharmaceutically prepared coal dust under bright and darkfield microscopes at magnifications up to 2000X and you will observe a black, totally motionless structure.

Now place some of the coal dust on the end of a metal probe and place it in a flame. It will heat up to near white hot incandescence. The next step is to plunge the white hot material into a test tube of **sterile** beef boullion or potassium chloride. There will be sudden implosive "fizzle-sizzle" and the entire solution will burst into a blackish cloud.

A half-hour later finds that some of the black cloud has settled to the bottom leaving the remainder a milky-gray in color. In a week it all settles to the bottom. Microscopic observations of what has settled show a remarkable change in the coal dust particles. They are filled with jiggling bubbles. Over a period of time the bubbles merge together and form globules

71.

that seem to pulse with some kind of energy and with an irregular rhythm. They have a positive electrical charge and they are moved in an electrical field. They absorb tissue dyes that are only supposed to stain living materials. The milky portion of the fluid contains little particles that can be cultured to produce fungus. The changes continue to evolve and some very small, fast-moving particles begin to appear in microscopic view. **Where did they come from?**

Ready for another? The most primitive or simplest life form is called the protozoa. Not a single biolgy book that we know of contains a description of the material composition of the solution in which the protozoa are found. They give no explanation at all about the origin of the most primitive of organisms.

Here is a direct quotation from a textbook on bacteriology: *"It is well to review the general characteristics of the various types of microorganisms ordinarily considered in the course of general biology. Water, to which some hay has been added, will abound after a few days in a variety of microorganisms, bacteria, algae and protozoa."*

That is the end of the statment and the end of the description. Not a single textbook we know of gives an explanation of how the organism got there. Where do the organisms come from?

Let's take some sterile water and fresh hay or other grasses and mix the two together and then inspect the water for microbes. There will be none. We will not see bacteria, amoebas or protozoa. If the blades of grass are scraped with a knife and the scrapings are placed in the water and then the water is inspected for the presence of amoebas and protozoa, none will be found. But if you leave it alone for several days, the "Wee Beasties" appear and you have bacteria, amoebas and protozoa.

Where did the life come from? The grass or hay was dead, it had been detached from its life support. The water was sterile. If the bacteria, amoebas or protozoa had been clinging to the grass or hay, they would have been seen immediately.

Time-lapse photography might help us. This is what will happen: The blades of grass or shafts of hay undergo an amazing transformation - a structural change. They lose their striations and become more and more vesicular (filled with little bubbles or vacuoles). The vacuoles begin to coalesce and gradually form a common membrane that incorporates several of them. After a few days this little mass begins to move with a rhythmic pulsing movement. Then it becomes different in that the individual components seem to move toward and away from each other within the overall membrane. Eventually, the movements become more pronounced and the glob appears to gather more energy. It seems to grow until such a time when it can leave the grassy shaft and float away into the environment. At this time it is a living mass, classified by the traditional texts as a protozoa. From this point on the mass can differentiate itself and other organisms appear.

HOW DO WE EXPLAIN ALL THIS?

When a dead organism undergoes decomposition, its individual existence comes to an end but the molecules of which it was composed may combine to form new living organisms. In the late 1700's, two philosophers, Buffon and Needham, contended that a special **vital force** existed in every organic molecule and that **living matter is composed of vitalized organic molecules which do not change but instead unite with each other in combinations that give rise to new life forms.**

Thus this vital force does not die when a complex organism dies because it resides within the organic molecules which make up the more complex entity.

But have we answered our questions yet? The questions regarding the life from coal dust and decomposing hay should be now self- evident. The rain experiment may be just a little vague since nothing was put in the rain water. But remember that rain water is not sterile. It has collected many particles of organic matter in its evaporative/condensation cycle. Allowed the nutrient media of water, these organic particles now begin to create life with an urge just as great as man's urge to create new life. The vital force will not be harnessed or stopped.

It should now be a bit easier to understand the basic principle of pleomorphism - that unique ability of primitive life forms to undergo form changes to adapt to their environment. In Systemic Candidiasis, yeast found in the gut readily transforms into a fungus as it reaches the internal body. It is totally impossible for us to wipe out this eternal vital force which will always be with us. We can destroy bacteria with antibiotics but we cannot destroy the organic material they are made of. As in a nightmare where two bugs are formed every time one is killed, we have created new super bacteria that our antibiotics no longer kill, instead the bacteria feast on the antibiotic.

The bacteria adapted to their environment and changed to become a part of it. **Does that mean that we are doomed to be overcome by the "Wee Beasties?"** No, but it does mean that we must change our attitude toward them. **We must discard the outdated and disproven "Germ Theory" of disease.**

COPING WITH THE "WEE BEASTIES"

Our last statement was based upon certain known facts that fly directly in the face of acceptance of the "germ theory." Let's take a simple example. If we were in a room with twenty people and a swab sample of the throat of every individual was taken, you would find that one hundred percent of the individuals had pneumococcus in their throat.

How many of them had pneumonia, the disease supposedly caused by the pneumococcus? Probably none. Why not? Because the environment was not right for the pneumococcus to explosively multiply and produce the symptoms of pnuemonia. That means that a healthy body just will not tolerate the presence of many pneumococcus - or any other dangerous organism for that matter.

Our whole approach to health should be concern for our internal environment. Are the eliminative organs working as they should? Are the digestive organs working as they should? Is the circulatory system carrying nutrients and oxygen to all the tissue cells? Is the lymphatic circulation open or are lymph nodes congested and swollen? Is your respiratory tract open and capable of supplying you with the precious oxygen you require?

The food you eat, the air you breathe, the water you

drink, the physical exercise you engage in, the clothes you wear, the social habits you have, your mental attitude toward life all combine to form your internal environment.

When you accept such facts as listed below, you will have taken a great stride toward the resistance to our biological adversaries which will always be there waiting for an opportunity.

1. Two ounces of unsaturated oil per day in your diet will depress your immune system more than a regular dose of cyclosporine, an immune suppressant drug.

2. The foods grown on the soils which exist today are woefully deficient in nutrients and charts demonstrating nutritional quantities found in such foods are untrue.

3. The Recommended Daily Allowances for nutrients are adequate to avoid frank disease but are not capable of producing a healthy body.

4. The use of food supplements are a must in the society we live in today if we wish to be healthy.

5. Exercise of one form or another is an absolute must for good health.

6. A goal in life is imperative for a proper mental attitude which is necessary for the production of the "feel good" hormones which make life pleasurable and disease resistant.

A Final Word

You have just concluded a comparatively non-technical, common-sense and clinically proven approach to a class of disorders that are epidemic in our nation today. You have the choice to agree with this program or you can continue to follow the edicts of the "school medicine" approach which tends to allow conditions to reach critical proportions before treatment is initiated.

Although our philosophy is firmly entrenched in the belief that health is our greatest wealth, it is quite sad for us to see how many quantify their treatment approach by dollars - "How much does it cost?" Ask any sick rich man what he would pay to have exuberant good health and you know what the answer would be. When you have health, you have everything.

Taking your health problem (large as it may seem) and breaking it down into smaller, treatable entities can only mean that you will improve. Building up the parts will inevitably result in a healthier whole. So go for it!

The Authors

About This Booklet

Kurt W. Donsbach and H. Rudolph Alsleben are leading advocates of the wholistic approach to health. In this booklet you will read the results of their many combined years of experience and investigation into the ailments of mankind.

Their advice is based upon looking at the disease process from a total physiological viewpoint, how the body interacts to prevent or allow malfunction.

You will receive concise instructions for home programs that you can use to create a healthier body and mind. Your understanding of the conditions that afflict mankind will allow you to prepare an adequate defense program before you are in an emergency situation.

**Printed and Published by
The Rockland Corporation**
©1994